FIVE LITTLE SUGAR BUGS

By Rachel Grider, RDH
Illustrated by Summer Morrison

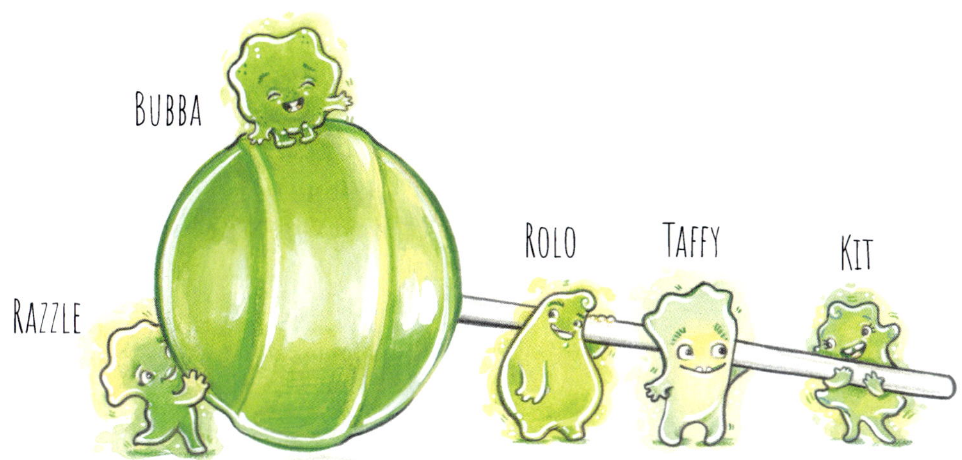

This book belongs to:

____

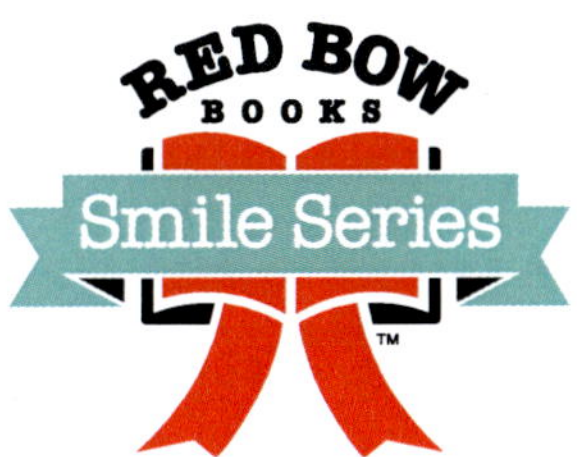

For Jim & Ivy - R.G.
Robin, Quinn, & Amora - S.M.

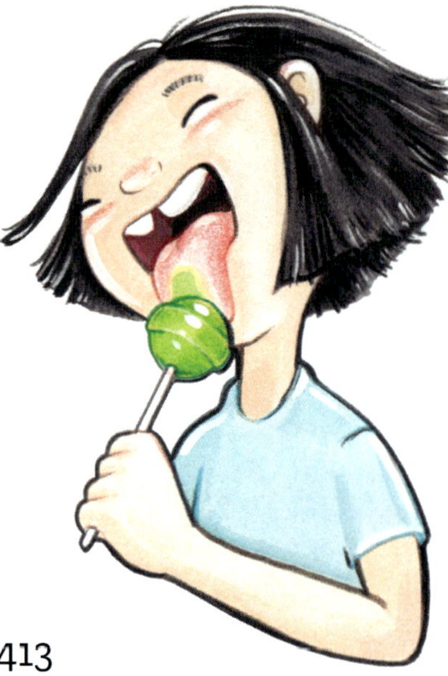

Published by Red Bow Books
The Smile Series

ISBN 978-1-7321568-4-5

Printed in the Untied States of America
Milwaukee, WI
Library of Congress Control Number: 2021922413

For more information, visit our website: www.RedBowBooks.com

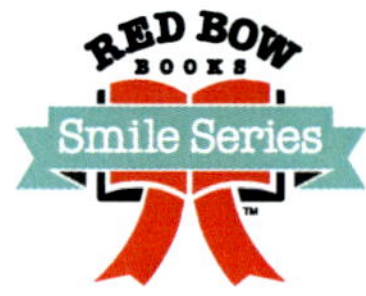

Making Little Smiles Brighter One Book at a Time!

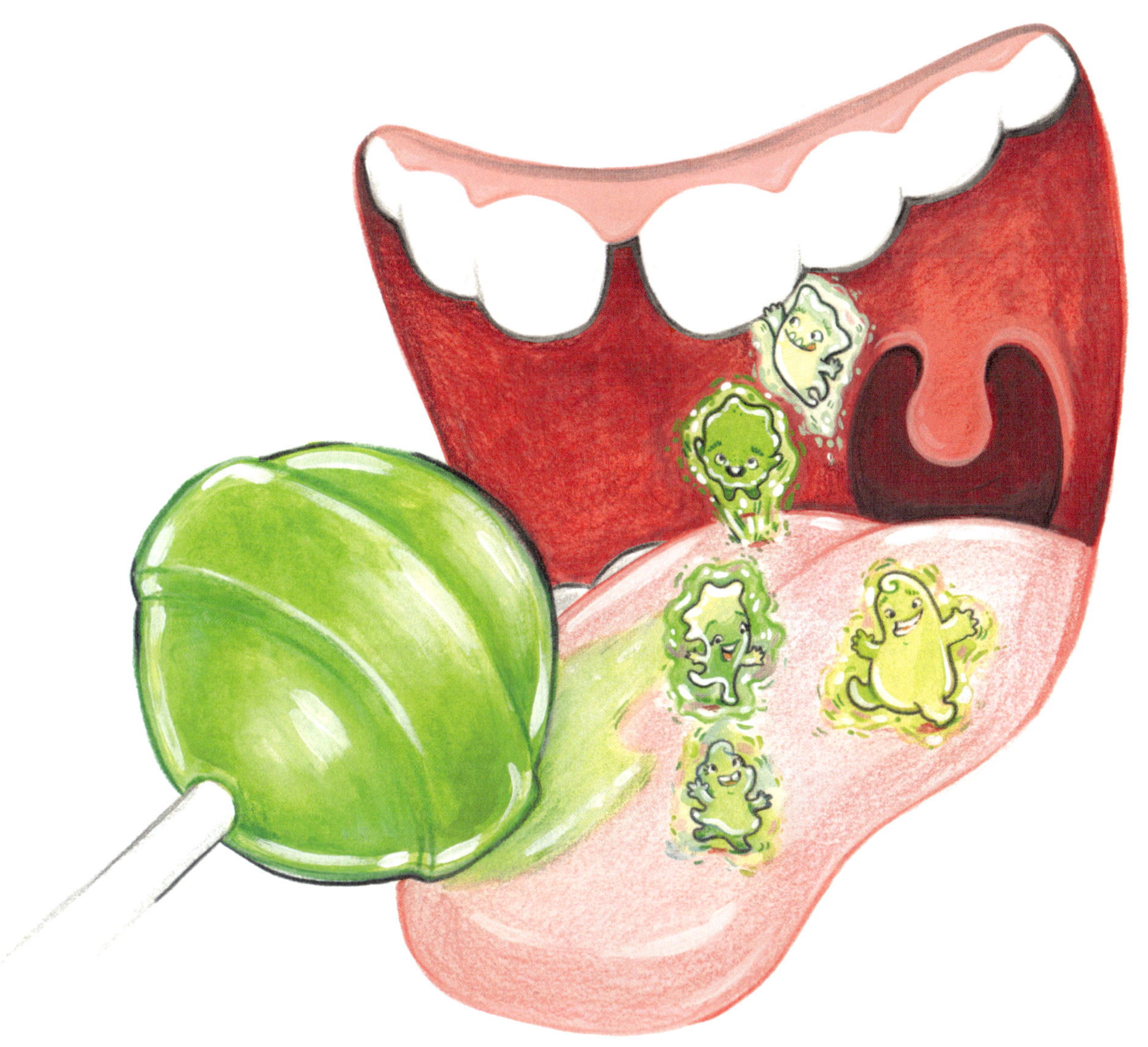

Five little sugar bugs were ready for the day.
On teeth and tongue and little gums they couldn't wait to play.
And play they did inside a mouth they hoped to call their home.
Then, one by one, each wandered off to look around and roam.

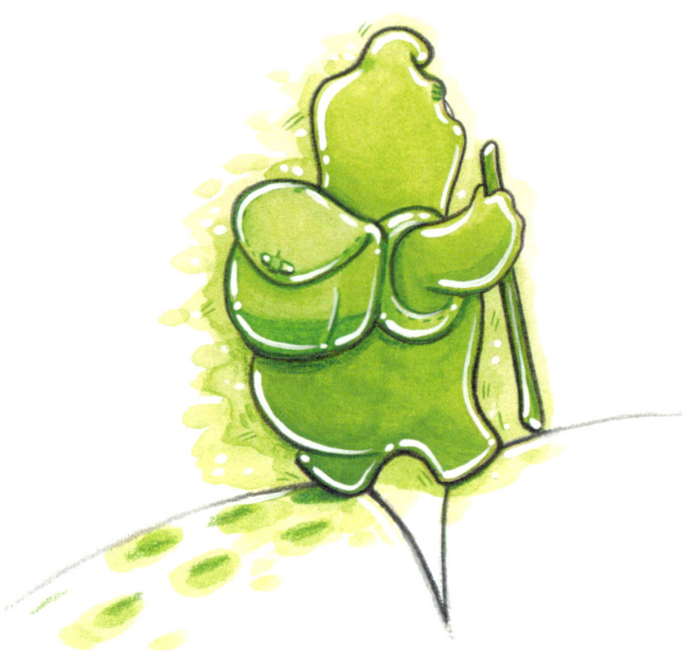

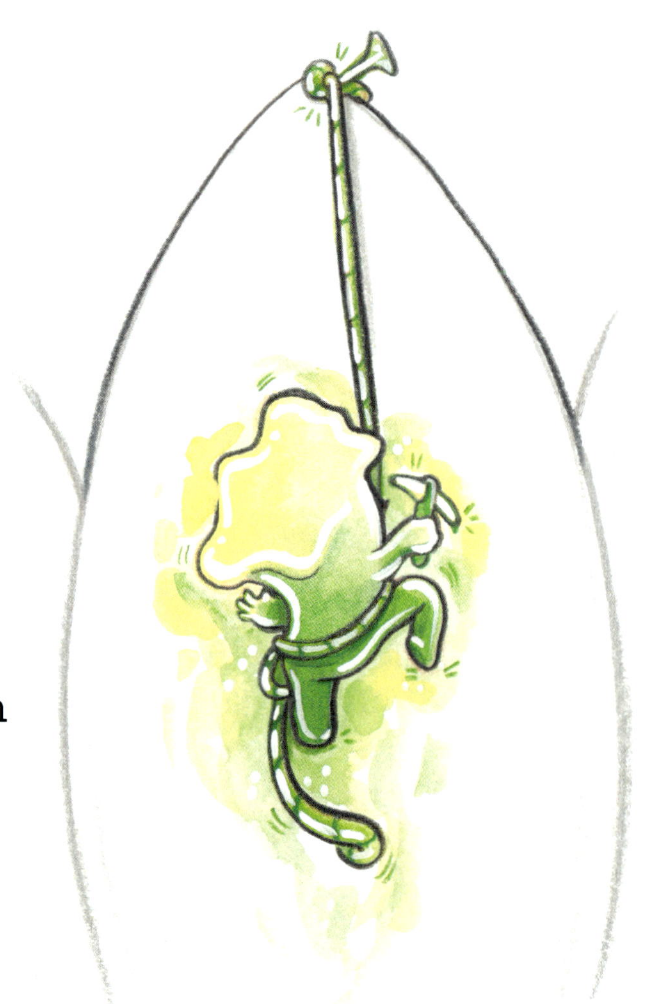

Rolo went off hiking,
exploring like a sleuth.
Razzle set out through the mouth
to climb the tallest tooth.

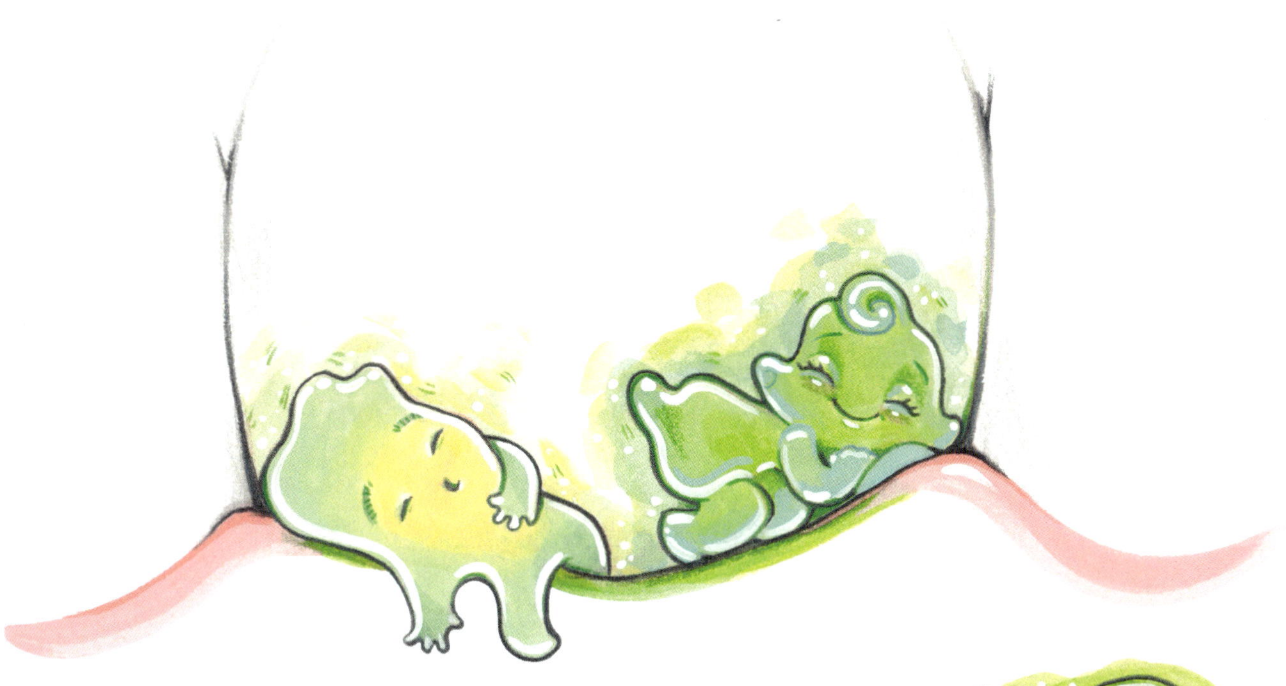

Kit and Taffy tucked inside the gums
and closed their eyes.
And Bubba bounced along a tongue
of great, tremendous size.

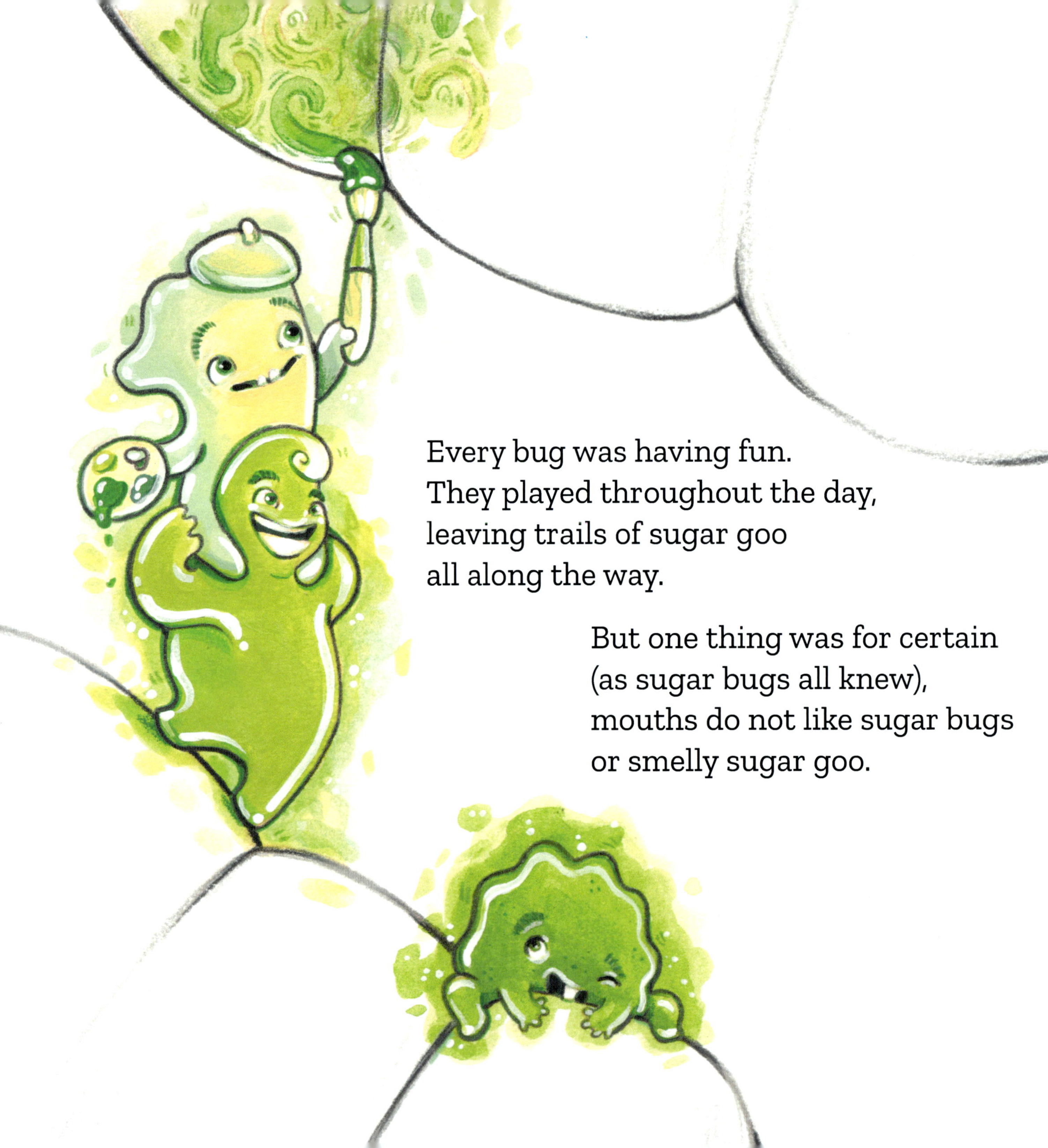

Every bug was having fun.
They played throughout the day,
leaving trails of sugar goo
all along the way.

But one thing was for certain
(as sugar bugs all knew),
mouths do not like sugar bugs
or smelly sugar goo.

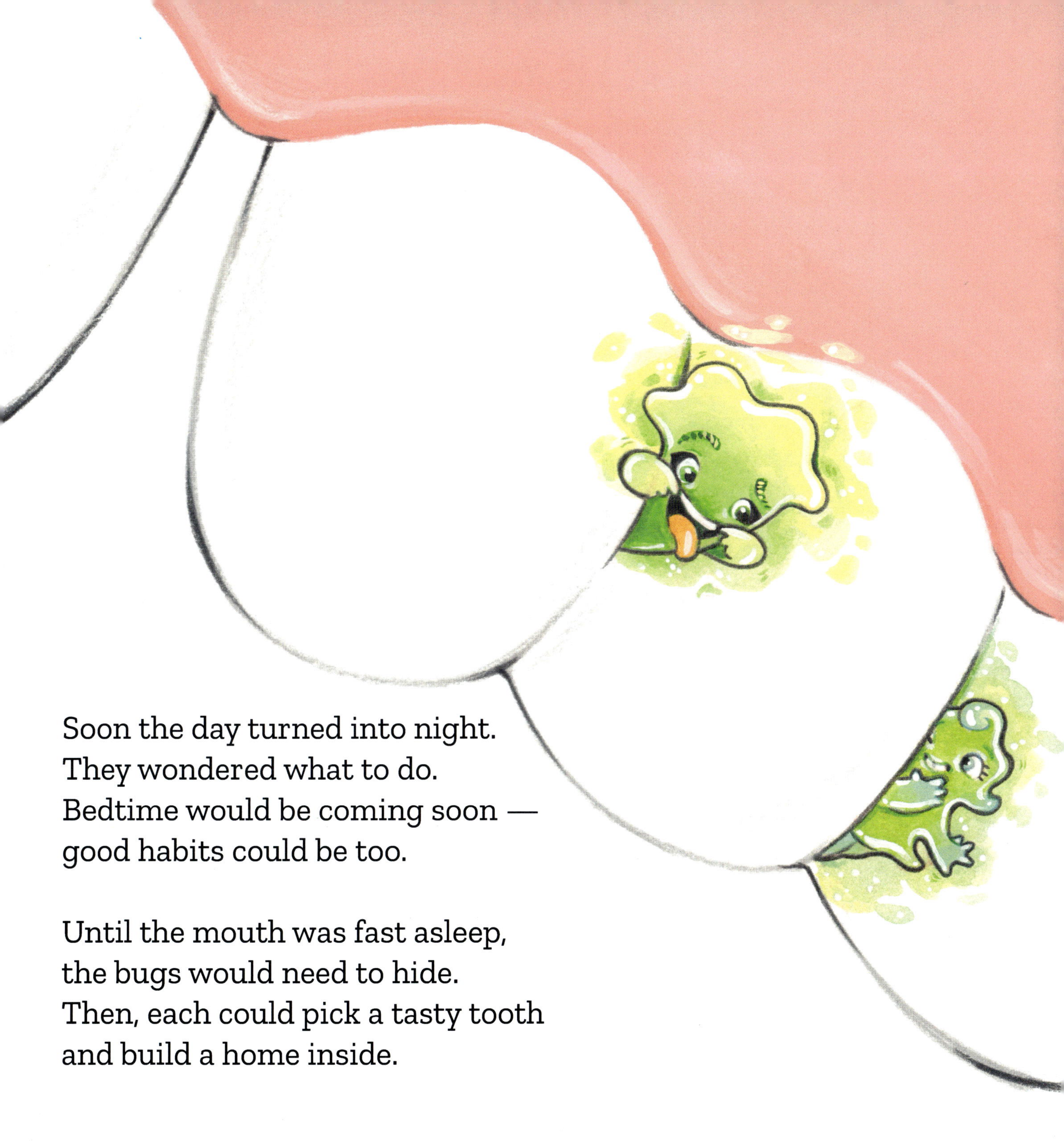

Soon the day turned into night.
They wondered what to do.
Bedtime would be coming soon —
good habits could be too.

Until the mouth was fast asleep,
the bugs would need to hide.
Then, each could pick a tasty tooth
and build a home inside.

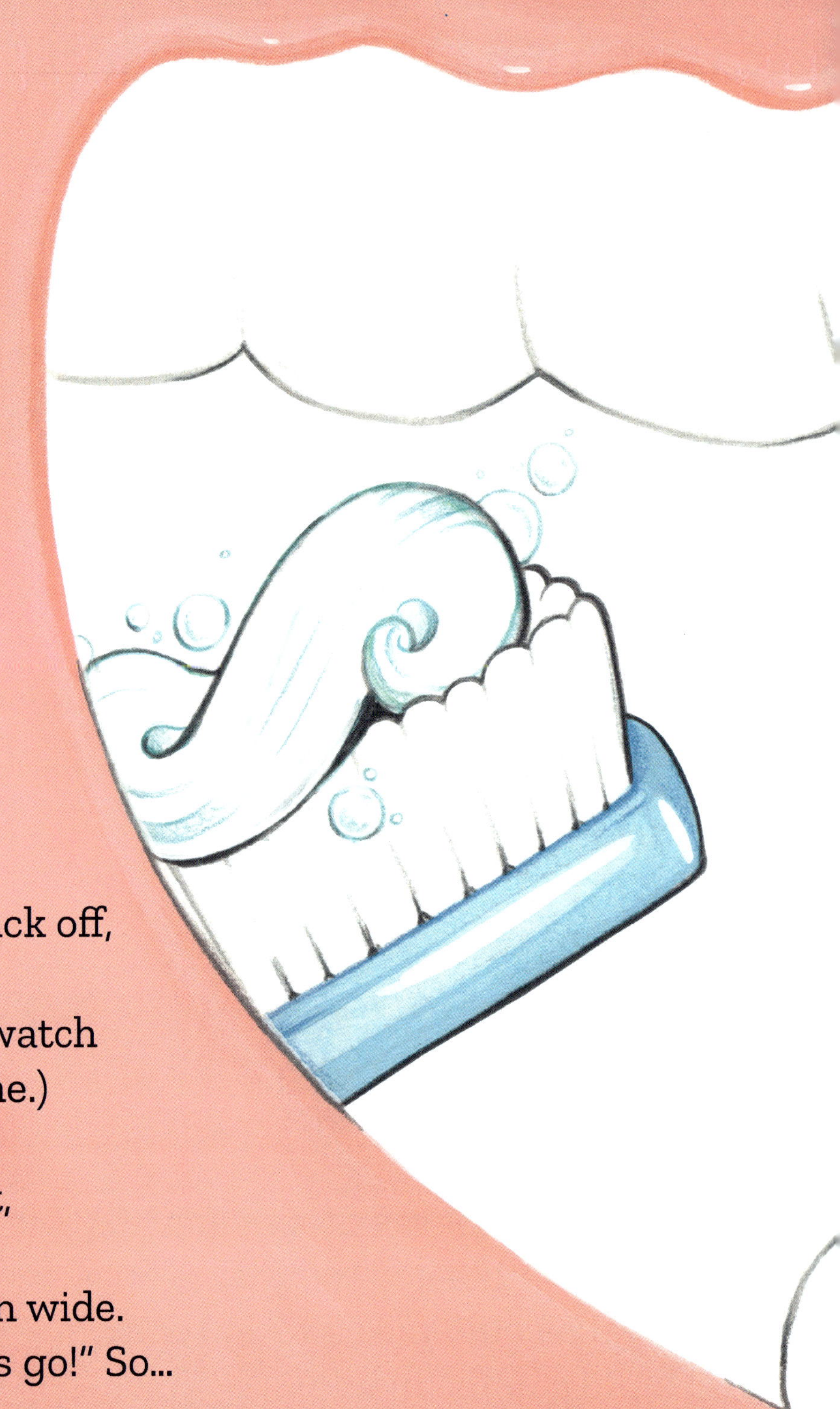

One by one, the bugs snuck off,
but Taffy left the line.
(Someone had to keep a watch
for brushing-flossing time.)

As Taffy took the lookout,
a light began to glow.
The mouth began to open wide.
"It's time!" he cried. "Let's go!" So...

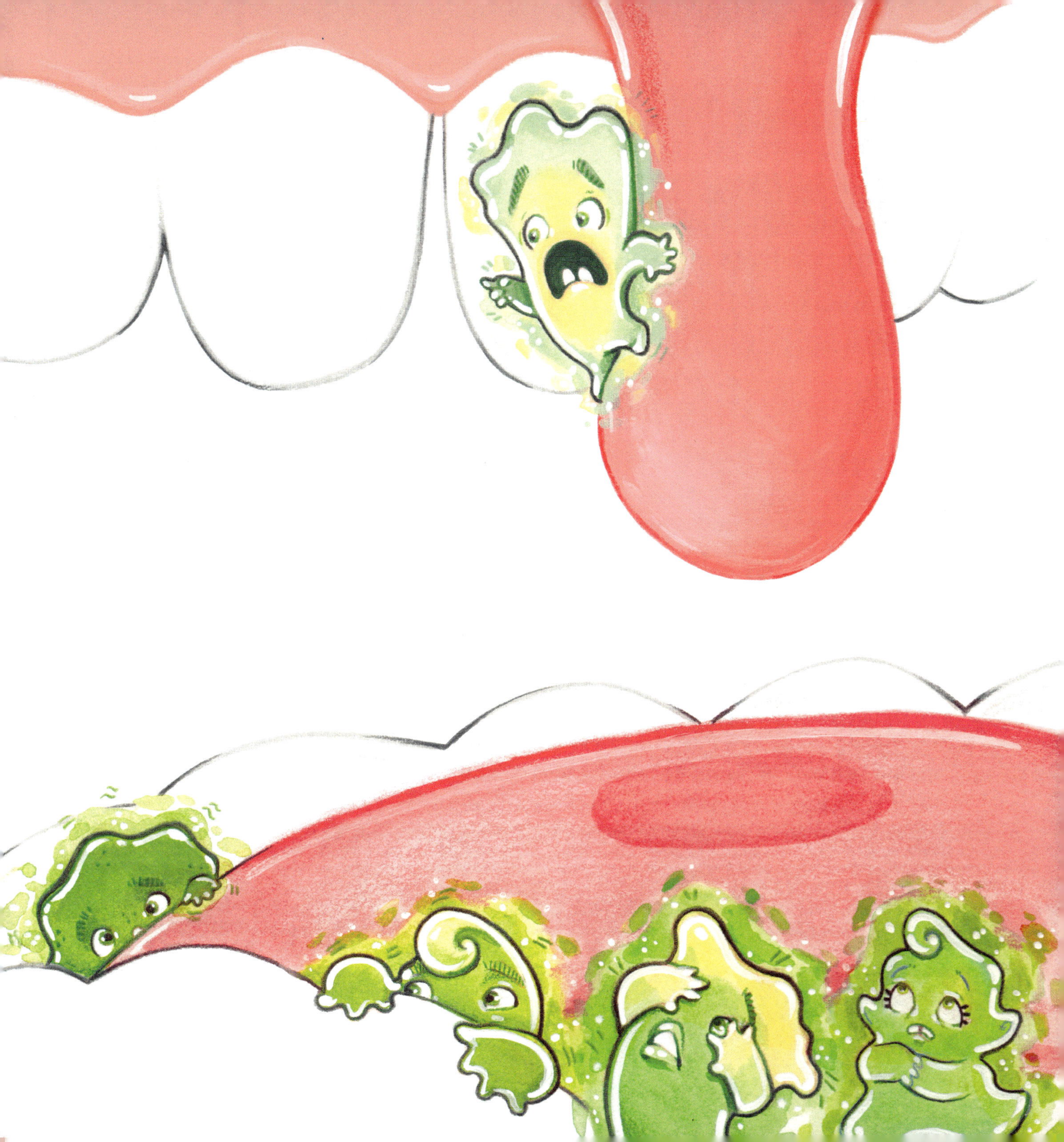

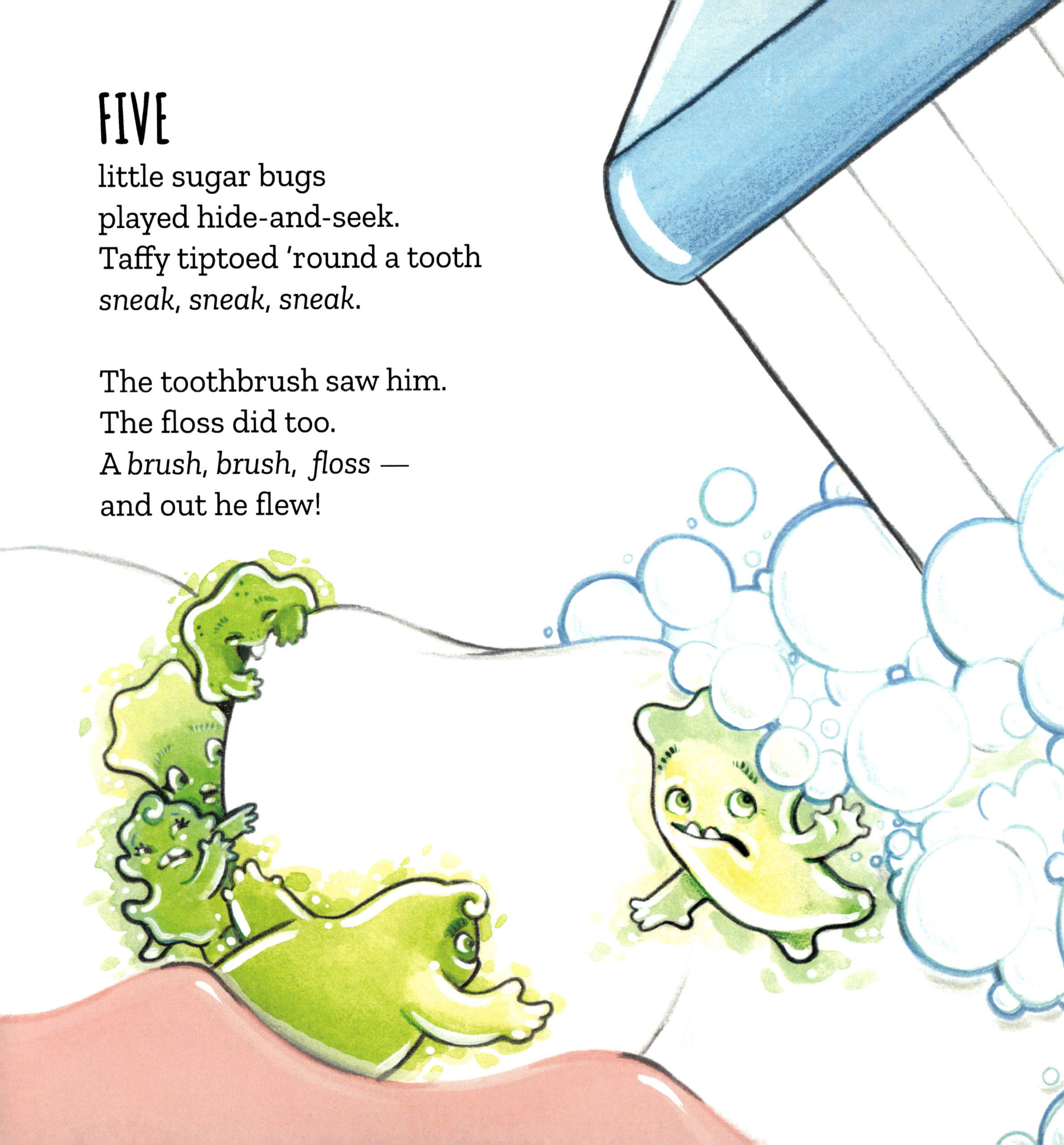

FIVE

little sugar bugs
played hide-and-seek.
Taffy tiptoed 'round a tooth
sneak, sneak, sneak.

The toothbrush saw him.
The floss did too.
A *brush, brush, floss* —
and out he flew!

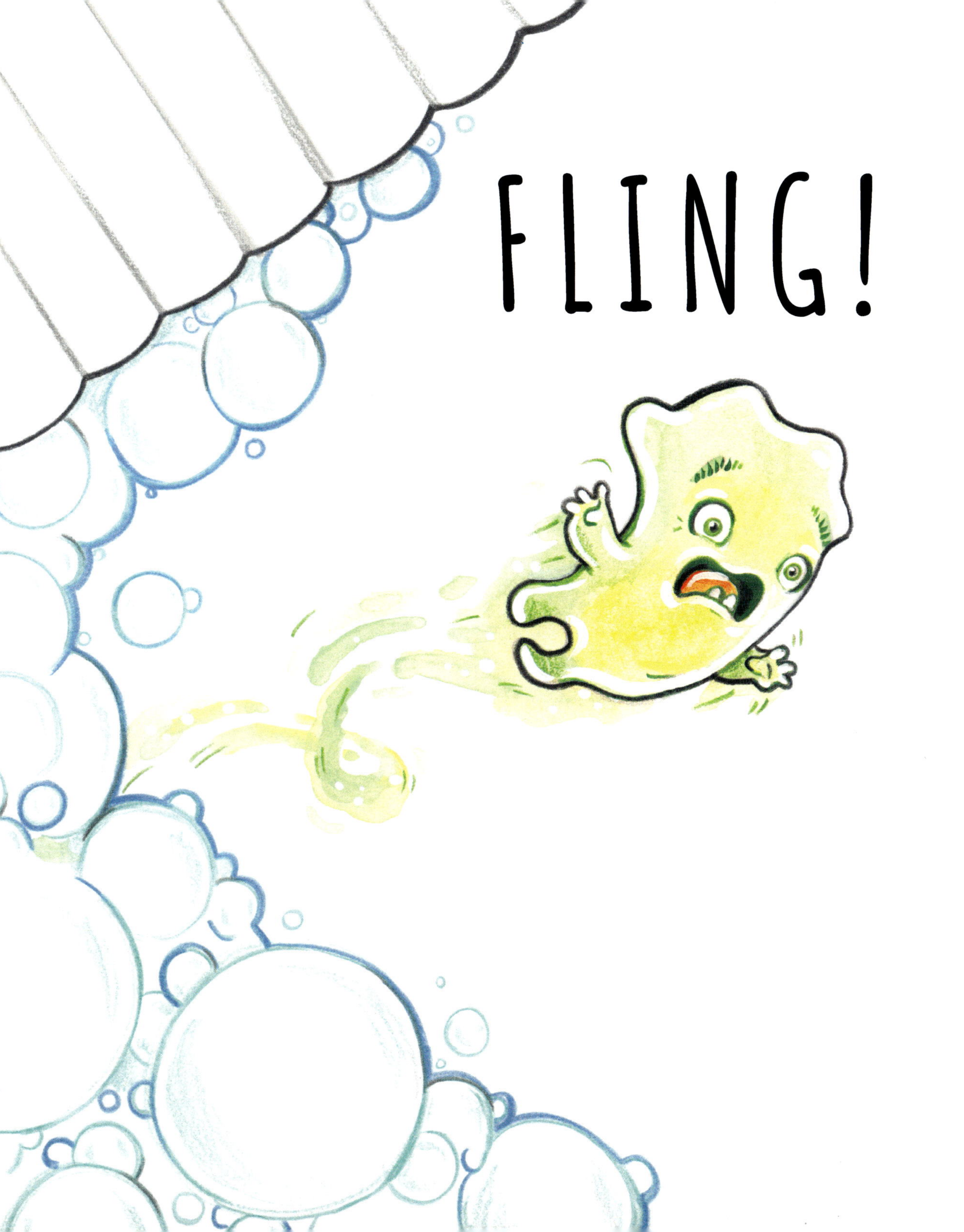
FLING!

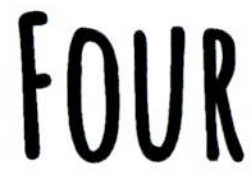

little sugar bugs
hurried off to play.
Rolo fell in sugar goo
and couldn't break away.

The toothbrush found him.
The floss did too.
A *brush, brush, floss* —
and out he flew!

FLING!

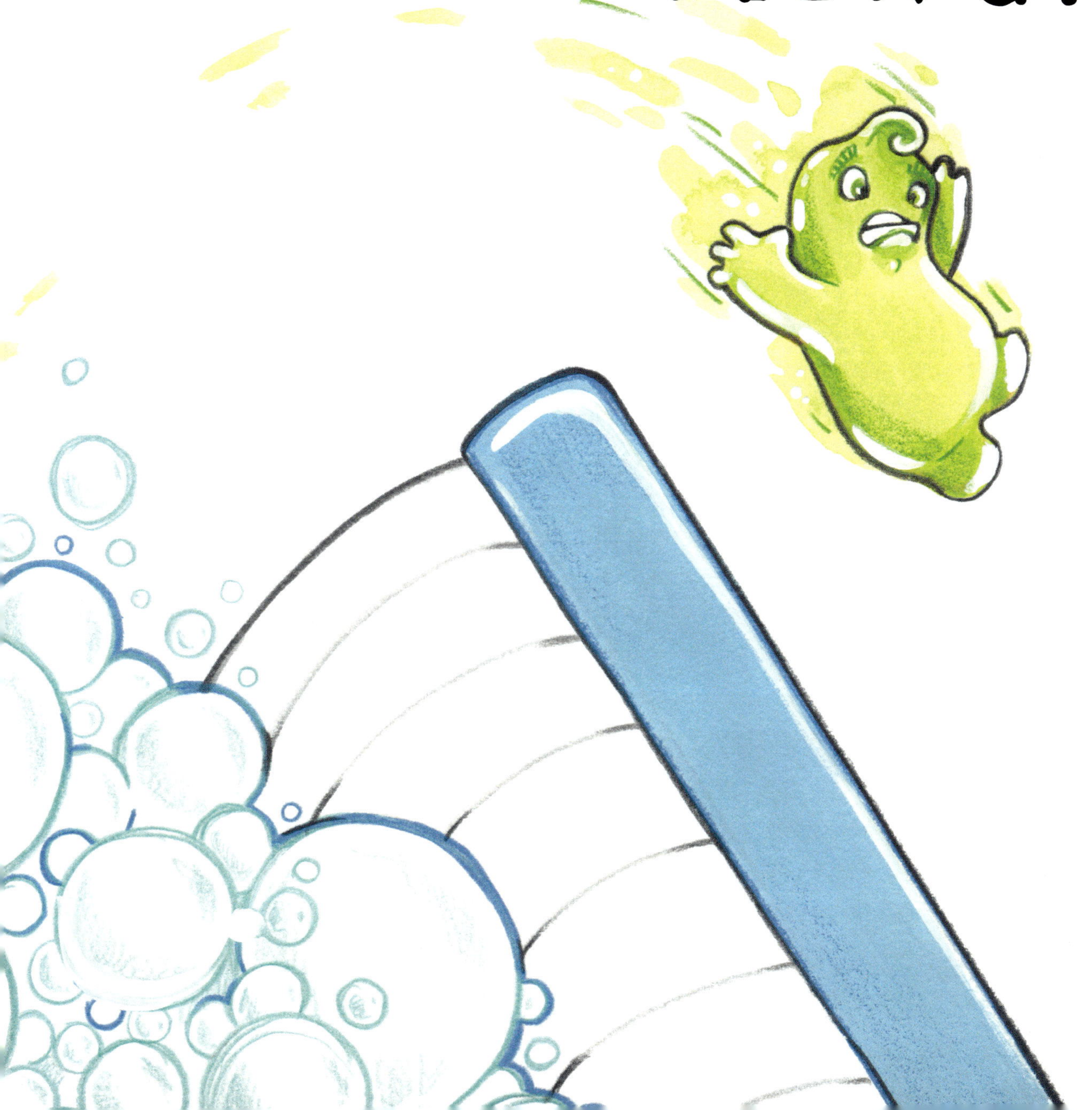

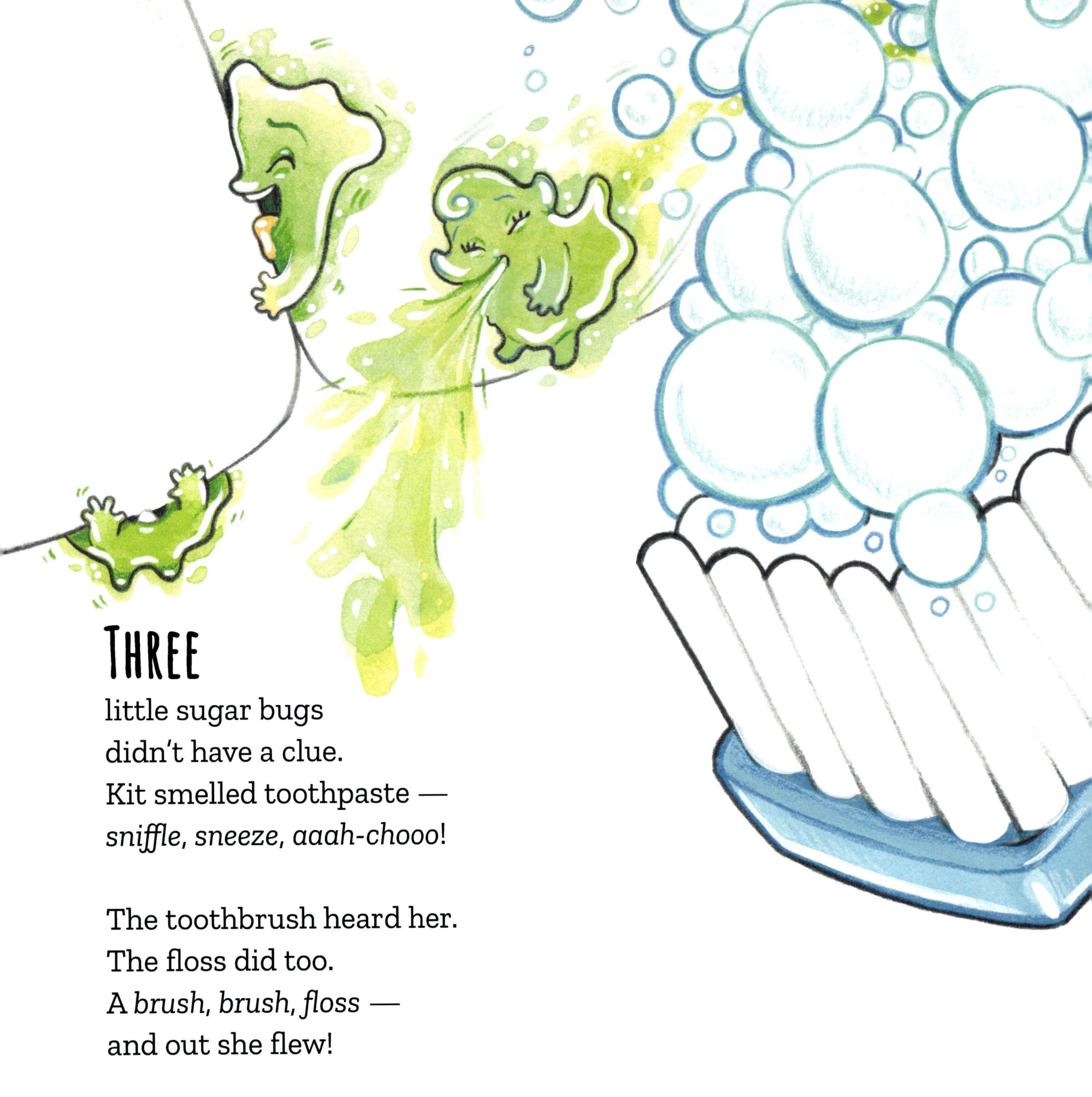

THREE

little sugar bugs
didn't have a clue.
Kit smelled toothpaste —
sniffle, sneeze, aaah-chooo!

The toothbrush heard her.
The floss did too.
A *brush, brush, floss* —
and out she flew!

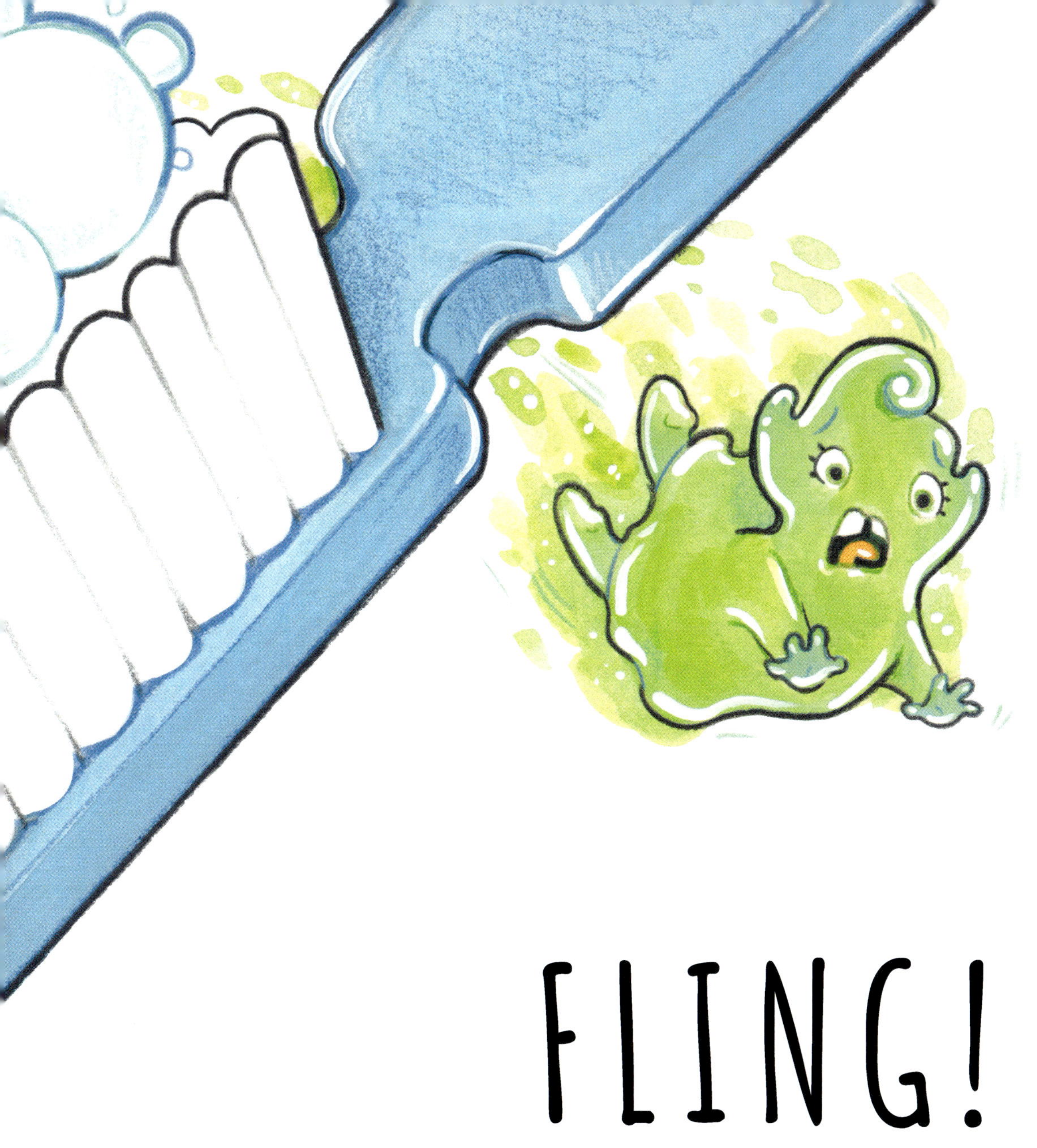

FLING!

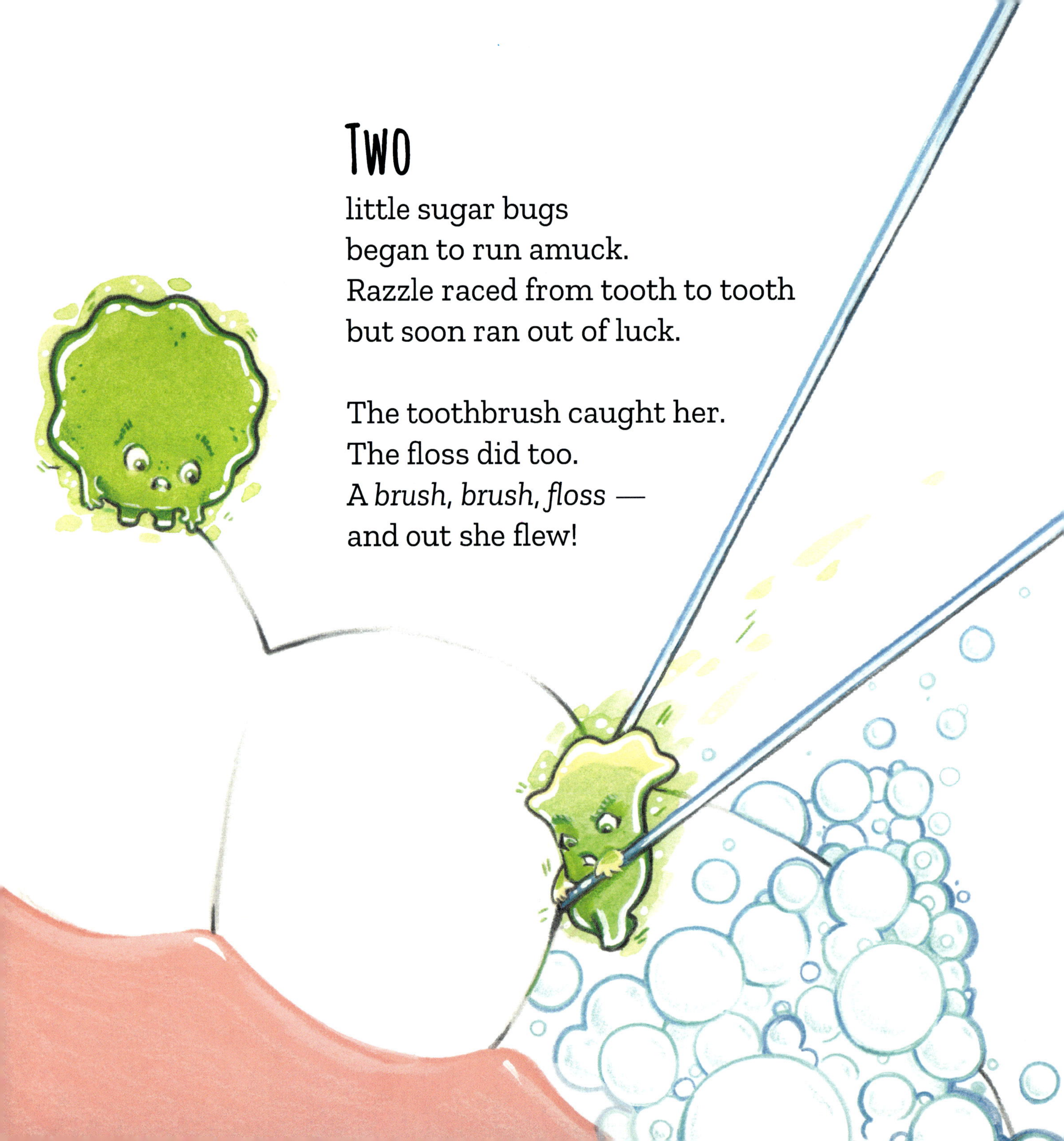

Two

little sugar bugs
began to run amuck.
Razzle raced from tooth to tooth
but soon ran out of luck.

The toothbrush caught her.
The floss did too.
A *brush, brush, floss* —
and out she flew!

FLING!

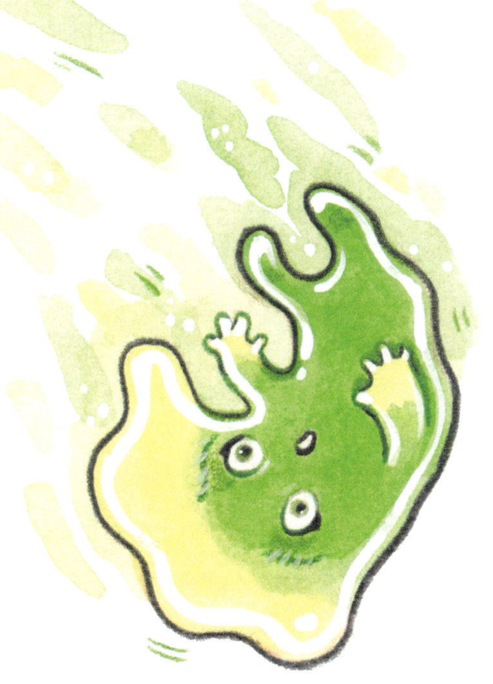

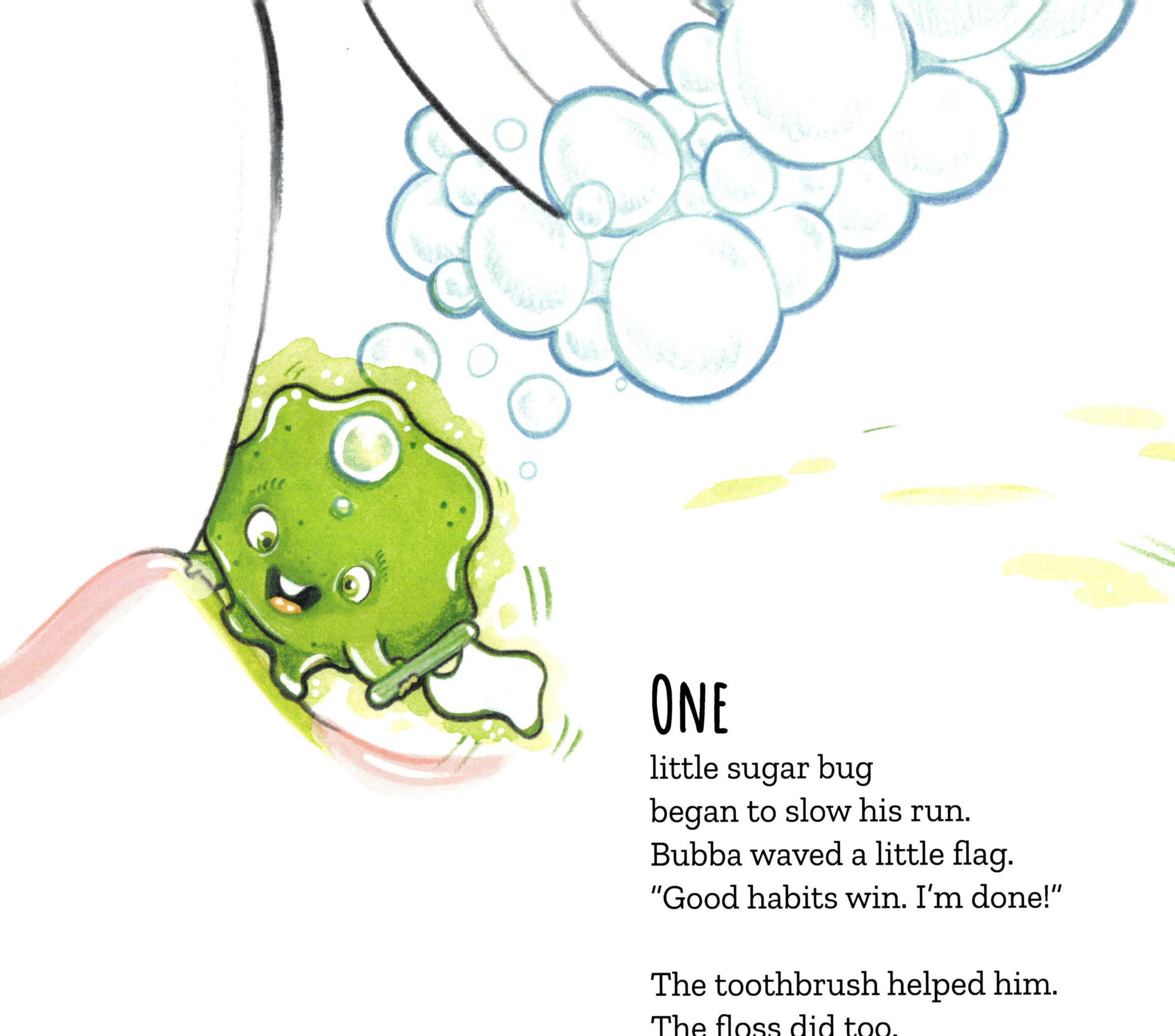

One

little sugar bug
began to slow his run.
Bubba waved a little flag.
"Good habits win. I'm done!"

The toothbrush helped him.
The floss did too.
A *brush, brush, floss* —
and out he flew!

FLING!

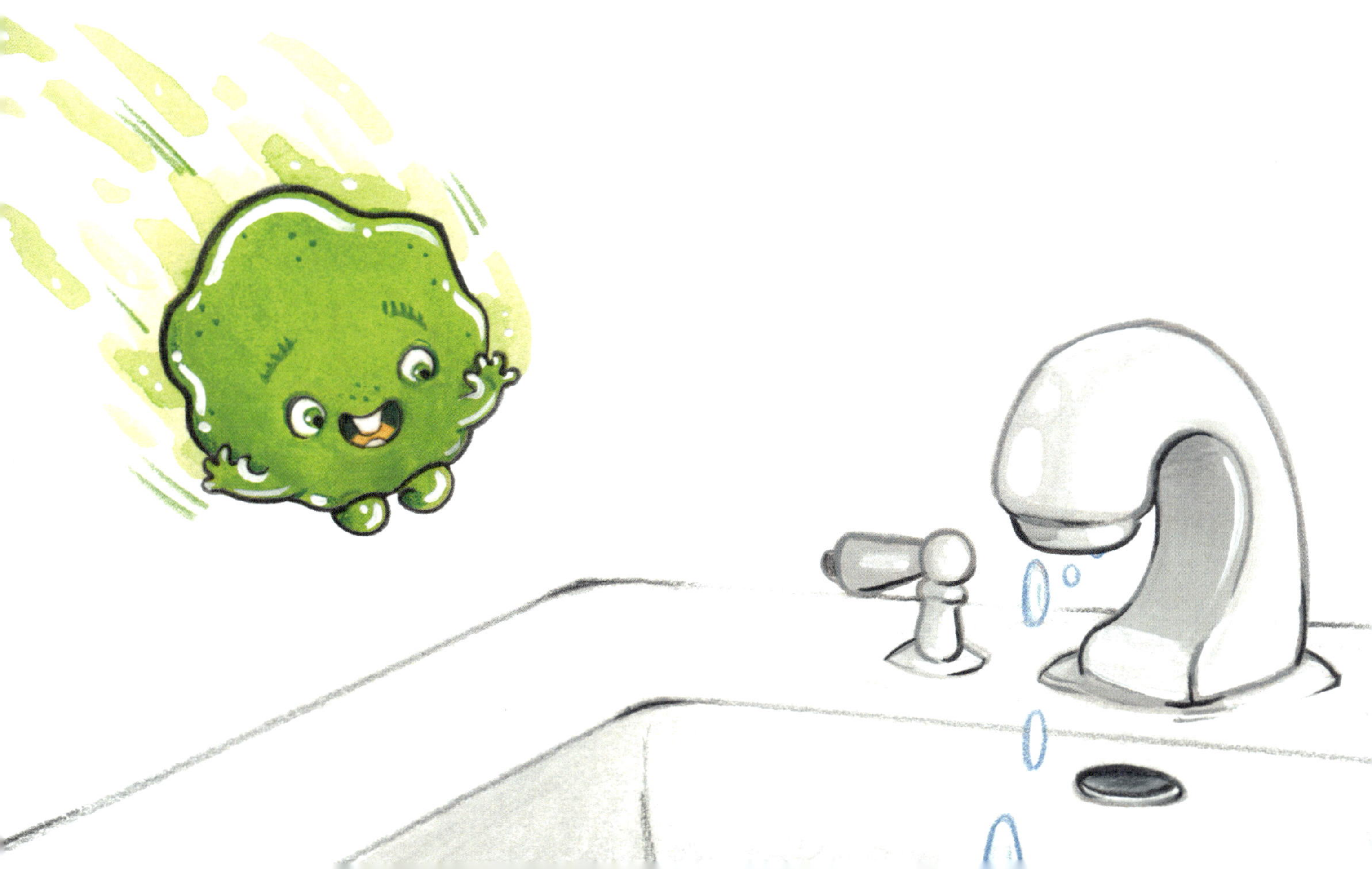

The five little sugar bugs
had landed in a sink.
(Being by a drain is bad
if someone needs a drink.)

Before the bugs could figure out
exactly what to do,
someone turned the water on —
and down the drain they flew...

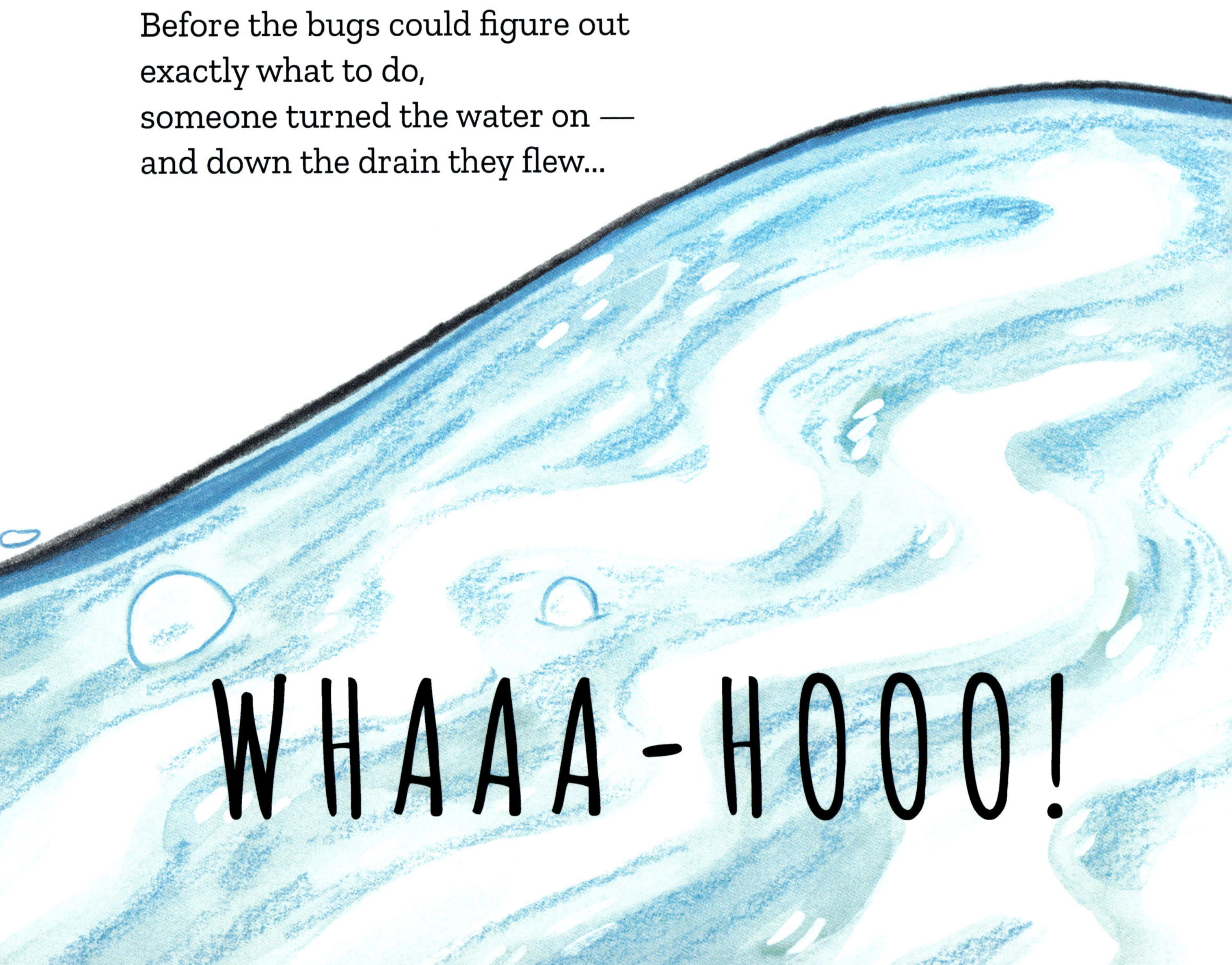

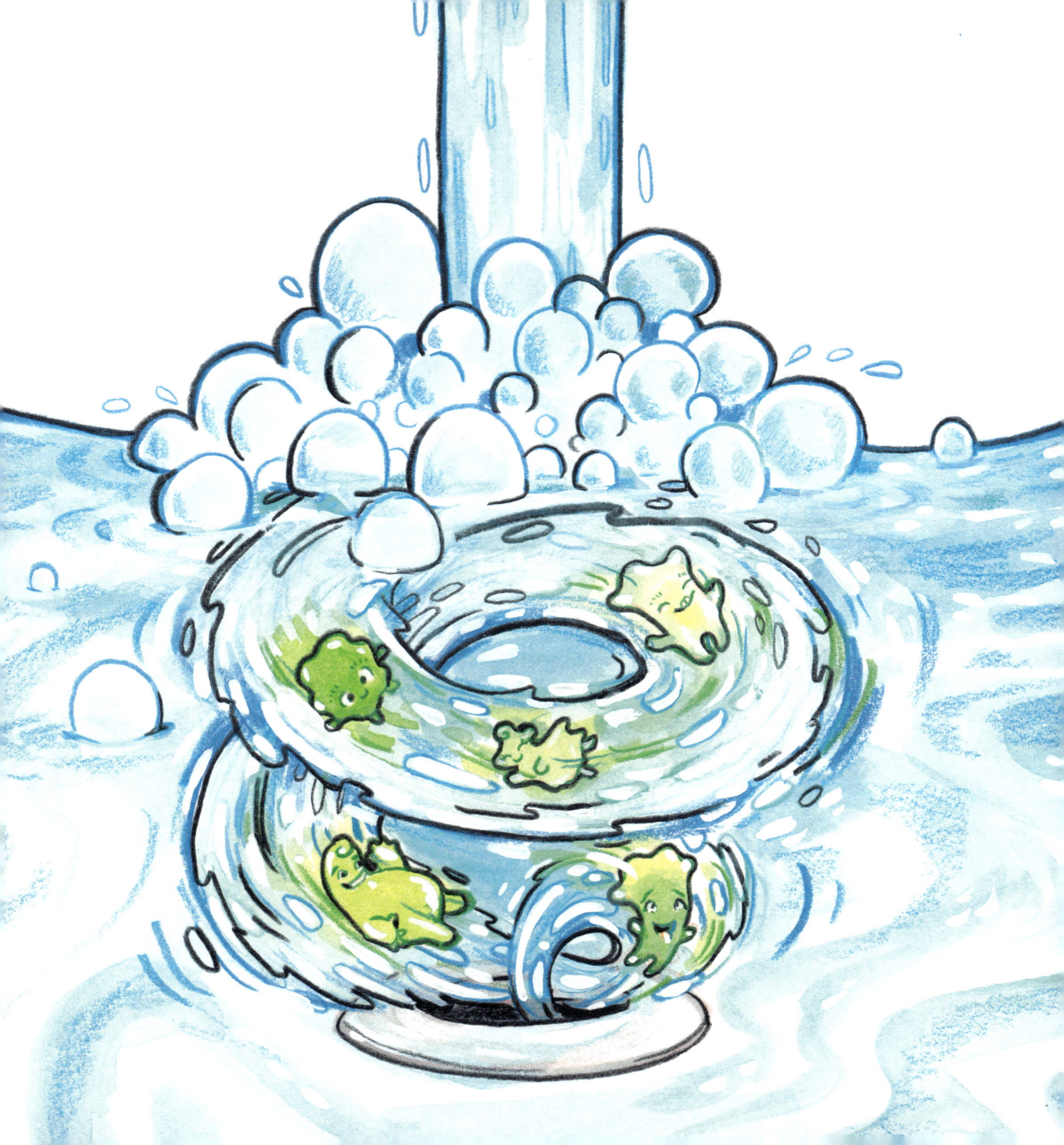

ACTIVITIES

Did you know?

Dentists recommend:

A rice size smear of toothpaste for babies and toddlers.

A pea size dab of toothpaste for kids 3 and up.

My favorite flavor toothpaste!

Connect It

What animal replaces some of its teeth every 8 days?

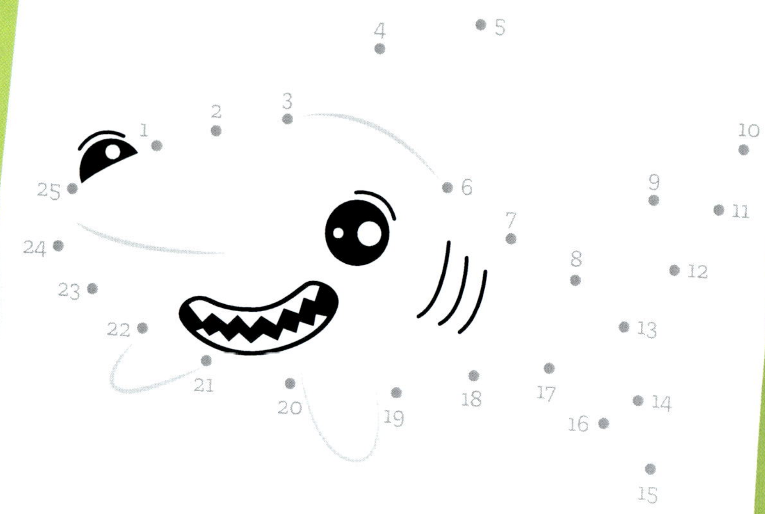

Answer: SHARK

My favorite toothbrush color!

Bubble Maze

Help the toothbrush follow the path of bubbles to the sugar bug.

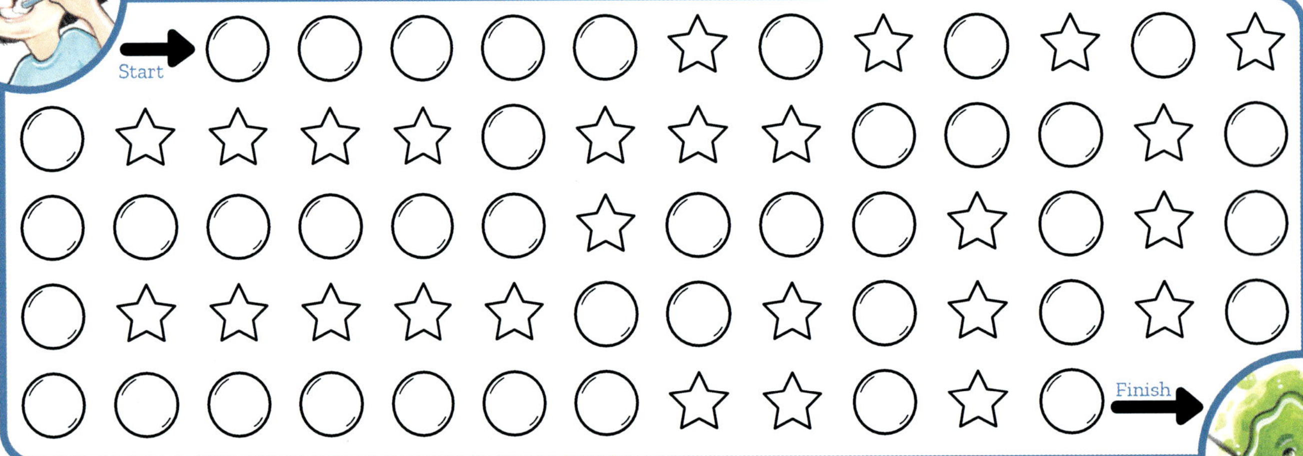

Secret Message

Answer: LET YOUR SMILE SHINE

Use the code below to uncover the secret message.

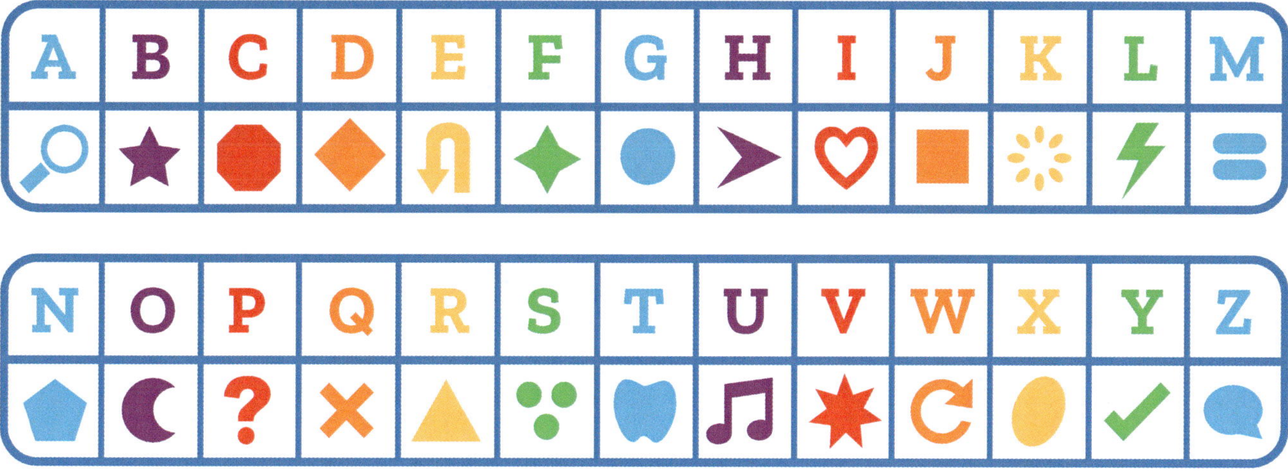

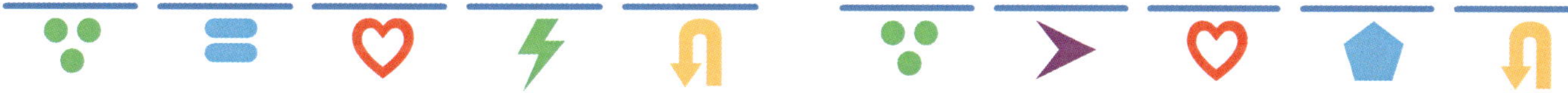

Sugar Bug Repellant

Brush for 2 minutes twice a day with fluoride toothpaste.

Floss every night before bed.

Eat whole fruits and vegetables.

Drink water.

5 Fun Facts

1. Plaque is a sticky substance that is constantly forming in our mouth.
2. Sugar bug is a fun name for the bacteria found in our plaque.
3. When plaque is left alone too long, it will stick to our teeth and gums.
4. Throughout the day, foods and drinks that contain sugar (or break-down to sugar) mix with our saliva and become sugar bug food.
5. When sugar bugs are full, they create acid. Too much sugar bug acid can harm our teeth and cause cavities to form.

Sugar Bug Sketch

What do you think sugar bugs look like? Create (and name) a sugar bug in the bubbles below.

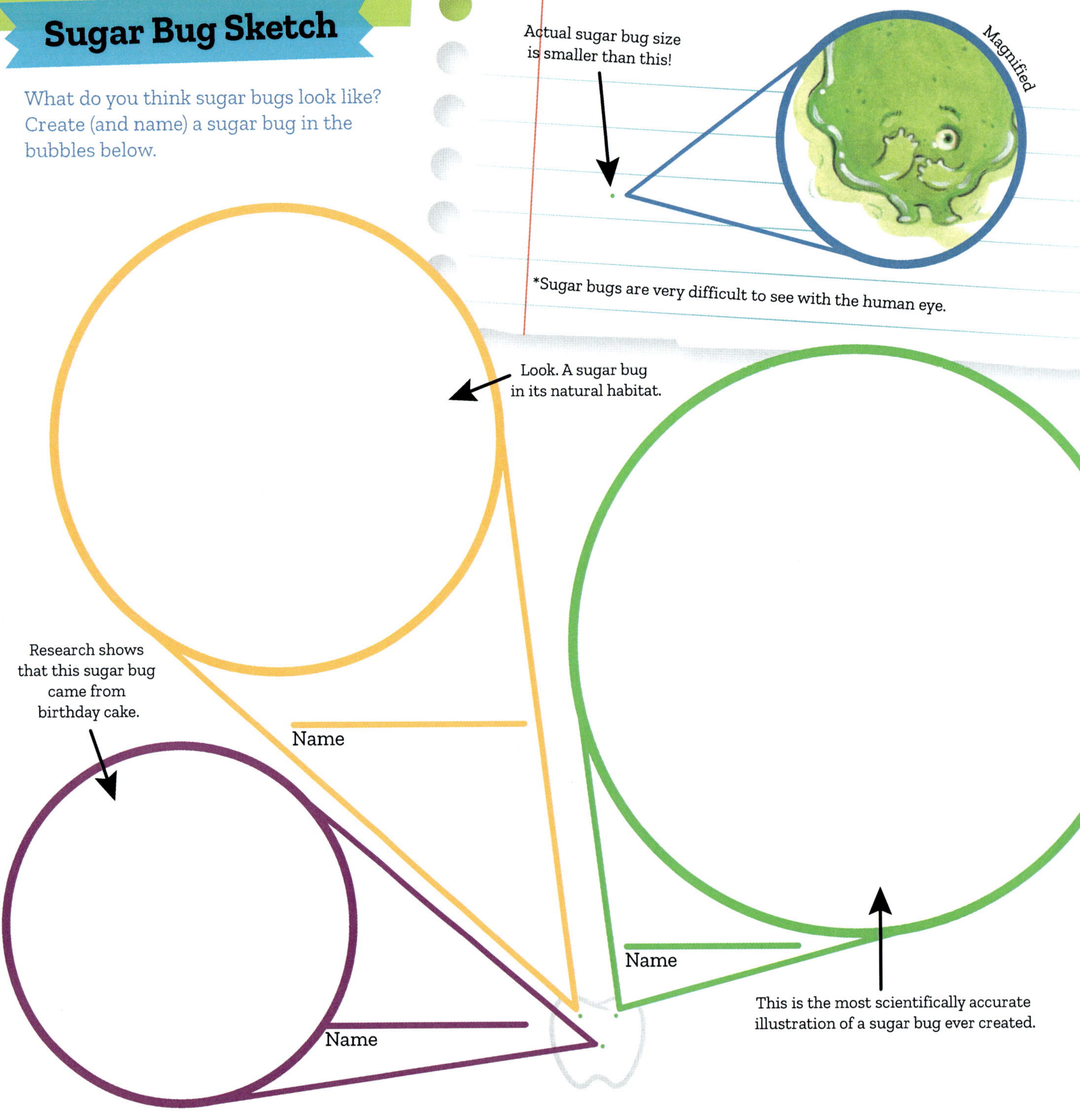

My Brush & Floss Chart

NAME: ______________________

WEEK 1

SUNDAY	MONDAY	TUESDAY	WEDNESDAY	THURSDAY	FRIDAY	SATURDAY

WEEK 2

SUNDAY	MONDAY	TUESDAY	WEDNESDAY	THURSDAY	FRIDAY	SATURDAY

My Brush & Floss Chart

NAME: ______________________

WEEK 3

SUNDAY	MONDAY	TUESDAY	WEDNESDAY	THURSDAY	FRIDAY	SATURDAY

WEEK 4

SUNDAY	MONDAY	TUESDAY	WEDNESDAY	THURSDAY	FRIDAY	SATURDAY

Made in the USA
Middletown, DE
29 March 2025

73468823R00017